I0091407

MEDITATION
FOR
BEGINNERS

HEATHER P PIPER

ISBN:978-0-6487761-8-5 First published by
Heather Piper 2023

DEDICATION

There have been many teachers in my life who have brought me to this book. My very early Yoga teacher in Sydney during the late 60s through the various mentors and teachers. The beautiful Buddhist nuns at the Rochedale temple who introduced me to that wonderful ancient wisdom and the modern gurus who will never know how much their words made a difference. And, of course, to my beautiful Yoga and Meditation students over the 23 years of imparting all this knowledge to them. To you all I say thank you - Namaste

MEDITATION FOR BEGINNERS

MEDITATION FOR BEGINNERS

MEDITATION FOR BEGINNERS

MEDITATION FOR BEGINNERS

CONTENTS

MEDITATION FOR BEGINNERS

MEDITATION FOR BEGINNERS

INTRODUCTION

I am tempted to begin with the standard statement of the day *"In these unprecedented times"* as seems to be the vogue at the moment. However, there has always been a time to practise Meditation and other relaxation methods in circumstances that an escape from the pressures of life is necessary. Times of war, illness, natural disasters and just the daily grind of work and family life can leave us in a state where the mind cannot relax, and so neither can the body. The next thing that can happen is the body begins to break down. Back pains, headaches, indigestion and other symptoms begin to appear that may have no obvious reasons for being there. Visits to the doctor or other health professional can have a diagnosis of stress as the cause and unless the stress is taken care of the symptoms will not go away, in fact they can get worse quite quickly. Medication will cover up these symptoms and may make you feel better for a while but unless you change the way you live your life the problems will continue to return. So, what can you do?

In order to maintain a healthy mind and body the most important treatment we can give ourselves is to be able to relax our mind as well as the body. If you live a very active life then your body may be in great shape but what about your mind? There are many new techniques available today that can deal with this and many classes that you can attend. However, sometimes the oldies are the goodies and I am going to give you some ideas of the various tried and true ways that have been around for millennia and some that have arisen in the recent past.

Relaxing the mind gives our brain a chance to stop. The continuous use of the brain can, and often does, end badly. Using medication might relax the body but it doesn't do much for the mind. In actual fact many medications given in good faith to relax someone who is always wound up for action can simply dull the mind, not relax it. Think about it. If you are always on the go and wind up exhausted at the end of the day would you just pop a pill at bedtime? Possibly. You might go off to sleep and wake up after 8 hours feeling bodily refreshed but what happens then. Your brain kicks in as you get ready for the day and off you go again. At the end of that day you pop a pill, sleep then wake up and off you go again. Your brain is ready for action at the first sign you are awake in the morning, but is it really? Your muscles begin to tense, your thoughts go straight to the tasks ahead and your Adrenalin kicks in. However, at the end of the week do you relax and clear your mind of the past week or do you go off to the gym, the shops or run around helping your children and other people do their thing? It is very important to be in charge of our mind if we are to enjoy quality of life as well as physical good health. So, when do you actually spend some waking time relaxing?

Relaxation can take many turns. You might like reading a book – like this one – or just sit listening to music. You might be a gardener or like to play with your children or grandchildren or you might just like to sit and do nothing or go and watch a sporting match. You are probably already relaxed in mind and body but please read on anyway, you might learn something you didn't realise.

I am going to talk about relaxation techniques you may have tried or may not. I have taught Yoga, meditation and Qigong for over 25 years and worked as a Lifestyle Counsellor. During that time I have come to realise that I still have much to learn. I used to try and meditate nearly every day, however, in my retirement I have discovered that my gardening, Qigong, Yoga and reading are also mind clearing, so I now tend to meditate maybe 3 or 4 days per week. We don't need to spend our lives sitting on a mountain top in Lotus position or leaving the world for a 4-week retreat, we just need to spend 10 minutes a day clearing our mind in order for it to be healthy and in good working order. I am coming close to the age my mother began to develop Dementia and my goal in life is to make sure it doesn't happen to me. My mind is very important to me, as is my body, and although I have some age related physical issues appearing I have a health professional or two who can assist me there. I would like to take care of my mind myself if possible. So, what about this meditation business? One of the main thing to remember is that you do not need to spend a fortune to learn to meditate. There are plenty of opportunities that are either free or low cost. You might be able to support a local Yoga and Meditation teacher by attending their class and you will be able to ask as many questions as necessary first hand. If you attend church or another organised religion you may find what you are looking for within that community. Whatever your path you can find it without travelling across the planet to sit on a very expensive mountain in Switzerland to listen to a hype by a self-styled Guru. That's not what it is all about. So please read on and hopefully become a bit more informed about this wonderful way of life.

MEDITATION FOR BEGINNERS

CHAPTER ONE

A BRIEF HISTORY OF

MEDITATION

It seems that meditation in one form or another has been around since man arrived on this planet. Although there is no actual evidence, it seems that most societies have had their own way of using a form of meditation. There is written evidence in the Asian continent going back thousands of years and some traditions passed down through tribal customs show forms of meditation. Shamans, Medicine Men, Seers, Priests, Priestesses and many other influential people use meditation to achieve their goal, whether that be spiritual, healing or contacting spirits and/or gods. Some use a steady beat of a drum or repeating mantras over and over to achieve the level required whereas others might stare at a crystal or flame. Just sitting staring constantly at something natural could have an effect of 'zoning out' of the real world. Whichever method was used it was in order to leave the normal thinking of the mind behind and reach another state of consciousness. In eastern religions there appear to be different forms of meditation, some where the eyes are open and some are closed and there are 'moving' meditations where the practitioner will dance or walk a certain path either chanting silently or aloud a mantra. Mantras are often in Sanskrit, an ancient language of the Indian subcontinent and usually consist of up to 4 lines which carry specific information for the invocation of divine powers. A Mantra can uplift and/or protect as the sounds can carry energy to various parts of the body resulting in a healing effect. Often the words have no actual meaning, it is the sound itself that does the job. Most folk know the sound OHM and this is one of the most commonly used sound. Just sitting quietly saying OHM out loud can have a calming effect on the mind. A commonly used mantra is OM MANI PADME HUM. Try it. Another way is the "Bee or Humming Breath" that is practised in Yoga. It's very easy and has an almost instant effect. To do this is so simple. Close your eyes, stick your fingers in your ears, take a deep breath and hum as you breath out keeping your mouth gently closed. The vibration that occurs is what is good for you. You can even do this one at work but warn your co-workers!

In modern times it has become popular for ordinary folk to practise meditation just to relax or to follow the ways of Buddhism, especially Zen Buddhism where deep meditation is a major part of the practise. Prayer is also a form of Meditation as it requires leaving the outer world behind in order to talk to the object of the prayer.

During the mid 20th Century the western world was introduced to meditation when Maharishi Mahesh Yogi taught the way of Transcendental Meditation or TM. This is a form of mantra meditation based on Hindu philosophy and is classed as transcendental because it takes the practitioner beyond the mind, beyond thought, to meet the spiritual self. His technique has been very successful since the 1960s in the West and is now used as a form of natural therapy. It did help to make it successful once the Beatles, especially George Harrison, told the world all about it. Scientists have found that during meditation certain changes occur in the body similar to what occurs in deeply relaxed people. *This includes slowing down of the pulse, lower blood pressure, a decrease in breathing rate and an increase of the blood flow to the fingers and toes.* The stress hormones drop during meditation and the level of lactic acid concentration in the blood reduces. They also found that with regular meditation the immune system is strengthened. Apart from the physical benefits meditation also aids in releasing stored negative emotions. It is a time honoured way of controlling the mind and during meditation there is a relief from the constant chatter and restlessness of thought.

PHYSICAL REACTION

During meditation the electrical activity of the brain moves out of the every day rhythm and consciousness or **Beta** rhythm and into the **Delta** rhythm which is related to the sleep state. On it's way to the **Delta** it passes through the **Alpha** state which is between waking and sleeping. During this phase the body gradually relaxes and the parasympathetic nervous system predominates. This is when the Fight or Flight response reverses. The **Alpha** state is a very pleasant state to be in. It has been likened to being awake in a sleeping body where a calm, clear, tension free feeling takes over giving the body a chance to rejuvenate and repair the damage to the nervous system that may have occurred in daily life.

People who meditate on a regular basis report an increase in vitality and concentration and a greater control over their lives.

If you wish to go further into the technical/psychological side of meditation there is much information available either on line or through your local library. However, I would like to continue with the pleasurable side of life with meditation.

CHAPTER TWO

CREATING A SPACE

Before starting your journey into meditation you will need to find somewhere to do this and we will call this your Sacred Place. This doesn't mean it is a religious place, on the contrary, it is **_your Sacred Place_**.

Find a space that will not be used for anything else apart from your relaxation. If you are also going to do Yoga there it will need to be big enough for your mat and your arms out wide to the side without touching anything or ending up with your head or feet under the furniture. This space can be inside or out on a verandah so long as you will not be disturbed by others (and pets) while you are within the space. If you are lucky enough to have some kind of covered space in your garden then see if you can turn it into your Sacred Place.

No phones, electronic gadgets or TVs etc should be in that space, although a CD player or other music device is OK. I don't recommend earphones for the simple reason that if you are able to completely zone out then the music should melt into the background not be stuck in your ear. If you can't move the above items out then cover them over when you are using the space. Make sure there is **no clutter** around. Clutter will only divert your attention.

The **ideal space** would be a spare room, part of a large verandah, part of a bedroom or even a walk in wardrobe, a sheltered garden area or even in part of a shed or barn if it is clean and quiet while you are there. Regarding the *area in your garden.* You will probably have seen, in a movie or on a TV show someone sitting cross legged on the grass, eyes closed, hands on knees in front of a statue of Buddha in a state of meditation. This is not a bad idea so long as (a) you aren't sitting in the hot sun, (b) no beasties begin to crawl up your arm or (c) the next door neighbour is not mowing the lawn. However, if you do have a nice closed in garden and wish to create a space then please also provide yourself with a raised 'platform' – about 10cm (4 inches) off the ground – to sit on and find a nice soft, wide cushion to put on it. I have one of these spaces created by my wonderful husband and it is the best place. However, we don't have close neighbours and my space is surrounded by bushes apart from a "see through" bush that lets me see the beautiful dam below our property. I also have no noisy neighbours using mowers. With an outside space it is not always practical to burn a candle or incense because a breeze may put them out before you have a chance to enjoy the space, however, if you are in nature you may not need anything more than the space itself. However, a statue of a meditating Buddha, a special flowering bush, running water or even a crystal geode can make your space special. There are many ideas on the internet showing how to create such a space, but as it is your space make sure you are comfortable with it.

If your space is indoors then once the clutter, electronics etc are removed or covered and you have the space required then it is time to **personalise your space**. Find a small table, a low cupboard or chest of drawers or even a low bookshelf, but if you haven't any of those then an upturned box will do. I will refer to this as your "altar", although an altar has connotations of a religious table and this is not what I actually mean. On the "altar" you can place an item that you consider sacred, a picture of a loved one, crystals or flowers and/or candles or essential oils. Don't put too much on it or you will have too much to look at and make sure the incense or oils are not overpowering. Too much lavender for instance can put you to sleep and that is not the idea is it? Please remember that **if you use candles or incense that they are extinguished before you leave the space and that they are on a non-flammable surface.** You don't want to burn the house down and sadly there have been quite a few fires in the recent past that were caused by candles that were left unattended. Fire alarms can certainly take the peace out of your meditation. I always open the window when I am using incense inside so it doesn't become overwhelming. Once the altar is done remember that you can always change what is on there should you need to or as your life changes. You might want to concentrate on something particular in the future and need to have an item there to focus upon. I will touch upon that later.

Next thing to consider is your **Yoga mat and/or cushion**. The cushion should raise your rear off the floor by a few inches so that your knees are lower than your hips. This will prevent you from tipping forward or backward when you are meditating. It is nice if you have a rug under the cushion and that your Yoga mat is to the side, but you might not have the space to do this so the cushion is on top of your Yoga mat. I have been using a Yoga mat made from natural and Eco friendly materials for many years now, however, they can be a bit expensive so just do what you can. It is not going to help you relax if you are concerned about spending money. Years ago my lovely husband made me a "chair" for meditation. It is low, wider than a normal chair so I can sit cross-legged on it, has a firm cushion and a low back support. The back support is important because when I am 'off with the fairies', as some folk call it, my back is supported up to the waist and I don't slump. This can also work with a two-seater sofa so long as it is firm in seat and back and if it is an old one with wooden legs perhaps you can cut the legs down or remove them so you are not so high off the ground. You will then have your purpose created meditation chair. It is very grounding to be close to the floor or ground but it is not necessary. I was in the meditation room of a Buddhist temple once and they had benches around the wall with firm square cushions on them big enough to get your legs up in Lotus position and these were at normal chair height. Excellent for those who can't get down on the floor for physical reasons. You don't have to sit on the floor to meditate. However, make sure that your chair or seat is not so comfortable that you fall asleep! That brings me to another point. Please don't lie down to meditate unless you are doing a special healing meditation (more later on this) as you probably will fall asleep.

Once you have created the space then it is good if you can **cleanse it**. This does not mean getting out the cleaning stuff and wiping it down – although if it is dusty or dirty you should do that too. Smudging is usually done with smoke as this will cleanse the space from bad energy or energy left behind by others. Sage or native flora is the best if you know how to do that but opening the windows and letting the fresh air in and if possible some sunlight is a wonderful way to 'cleanse' a space. You may have seen smoking ceremonies carried out by 1st Nations people before events on their land. This is cleansing with smoke. I have known of someone allowing the moon to shine in on a full moon but this will depend on which way your window faces.

It's OK if others enter your sacred space but **ask them to respect its purpose**. Children, cats and dogs seem to find sacred spaces calming and you might find your moggie or furry friend curled up on your cushion or a toddler fast asleep. Usually when I go down to my meditation garden I find that a wallaby or two has spent the night on the platform (obvious by the gifts they leave behind). That's OK. Their innocent energy will not create any problems with the space but it's not there for them to permanently take it over as a bed. If necessary pick up your cushion etc when you have finished with it.

Now you have your sacred space. Use it for Yoga, meditation, reciting mantras or chanting but also for if you need a quiet space to read or just get away from a busy household. If this space is all yours and there is enough room, an old fashioned bean bag is a wonderful addition for reading and quiet time. It will wrap itself around you which is always comforting. A light blanket or throw is also a handy thing to have on hand.

CHAPTER THREE

MANTRAS AND

OTHER CHANTS

If you would like to include the use of Mantras or chanting with your meditation there are many kinds that can be used. Different organised religions have basic mantras although the most common are connected to Hinduism. A Mantra is usually a verse, generally one or two lines which carry a specific information for the invocation of divine powers or just to being peace to the mind of the practitioner. A Mantra can uplift and protect. The combination of various letters are sounds and can carry specific spiritual potential which can unfold in the physical and non-physical (ie. Aura) bodies. The sound waves released by repeating the mantra can awaken power centres within the body and the repetitive uttering or chanting of the mantra helps mental, physical and spiritual health.

Mantra Meditation is a simple relaxation technique. There are no mysteries or secrets. Many mantras use the sound OHM. This is a word with no actual meaning so does not provoke any association with religion. In itself OHM can induce relaxation. Close your eyes and after about a minute of gentle breathing softly speak OHM as you breath out and keep repeating it with your voice becoming softer with each time. Eventually the word will only be in your mind. It is a powerful word that with regular use can induce a deep meditative state. The word should not be used in fun to make fun of meditation as it is powerful in itself.

To practise chanting OHM start with an inhale, as you breathe out imagine the word coming from the back of your throat as "OH" as you bring the word forward you close the mouth to create the sound "M". The more you practise the more the energy is invoked. There is a belief that it is the first sound from the beginning of the Universe. Whatever the origin it is a powerful and beautiful sound to invoke either out loud or silently in your mind.

Another simple but effective chant is the letter "M". Just repeating it over and over with your eyes closed in a quiet place will invoke a peaceful response. Try it.

MANTRAS FOR DIFFERENT

SPIRITUAL BELIEFS

Various spiritual beliefs have Mantras associated with their particular beliefs and some have been chanted for many centuries. However anyone interested in a particular creed can chant these in their own Sacred Space.

Some easily learned Mantras associated with Buddhism and Hinduism are as follows:

GAYATRI MANTRA

OM BHOOR, BHUVAHA SWAHA, TAT SAVITUR, VARENIYAM, BHARGO DEVASYA, DHEEMAHI DHIYO, YO NAHA, PRACHODAYAT

Mantra for peaceful thoughts:

OM MANE PADME HUM (Om, jewel in the lotus, hum)

The Great Peace Mantra:

Om Shanti, Shanti, Shanti (Om Peace, Peace, Peace) for personal and global peace.

CHAKRA MANTRAS:

Root Chakra – LAM

2nd Chakra – VAM

3rd – RAM

4th – YAM

5th – HAM

6th – KSHAM

7th – OM

CHRISTIAN MANTRA:

Lord Have Mercy, Christ Have Mercy or:

Kyrie, Eleison, Christe, Eleison (Lord have mercy upon us, Christ have mercy upon us)

ISLAMIC:

Bismillah, Al-Rahman, Al-Rahin (The name of Allah the Compassionate, the Merciful

HEBREW:

Shalom (repeated 6 times in a whisper)

There are many more from Ancient Egyptian to modern beliefs mantras have been used for centuries, millennia and beyond. Find one that suits you and explore the possibilities.

CHAPTER FOUR

PRACTISING

MEDITATION

There are a variety of ways meditation can be used, the one most widely known in the modern world is for relaxation. However, that is only a small part of what meditation can be used for. It is important to remember that meditation is a discipline. Like any disciplines when you first begin there can be difficulties. The first may be finding the regular time to practise and being able to find your quiet place away from the noises and interference of daily life. There is no point trying to meditate at work or in the living room at home when there are other people there as everything around you will cause distraction. The next reason to meditate may be learning to sit still and relax the body. Fidgeting will not bring on a quiet mind it is necessary to get comfortable first then settle the mind. Quietening the mind can be hard to learn for some whereas it may come easily to others. If you are a thinker more than a doer then this might be the hardest thing you have to do, so persist and it will come. As soon as you sit down your mind will be thinking of how you are going to quieten it. This is called the Monkey Mind in Buddhism and is not always easy to control. But you can learn to control it.

I can assure you, and people who know me will testify to the fact that if I can learn to quieten the Monkey Mind then most people can! It can sometimes help to go into a garden or sit on a verandah to release your mind from other thoughts. Even a nice cup of chamomile tea can help.

I will try to take you through the variety of meditations beginning with basic relaxation varieties. Please, find a quiet place to sit where you are comfortable, put your phone on silent (or turn it off) and remove it from your space along with other electronic devices (apart from your music) and read on.

CHAPTER FIVE

BEGINNING THE

JOURNEY

If you have never ventured into meditation before it's not a bad idea to try and find a group that is practising relaxation meditation and join in for a couple of sessions, Yoga classes are good for this. Organised meditation is usually led by someone who talks the group through the first stages, then you spend some time in silence before being brought back to the present. However, if you are unable to do this then please try the following.

With *your sacred space ready, make sure you aren't going to be disturbed* (if possible) and take a seat. Please don't lie down, you might nod off. In a comfortable position, cross legged or not with your back softly straight, place your hands gently on your knees, thighs or folded together in your lap. Close your eyes. Take several deep slow breaths – in through your nose and out through your nose. Begin to allow the breath to become natural and flowing and allow any thoughts that arise to drift away. Recognise them as thoughts but don't dwell on them. This might take some time at first but don't force it. If you can spend 5 minutes the first time then that is OK, you will be able to extend that time as you practise. After a while you should be feeling relaxed and that is the idea. If you need to then open your eyes but keep them soft and look at the items on your altar or nature for a while. If you feel like closing your eyes again then do so, this is good, but don't worry if you feel restless, as this is normal until you get used to leaving the world behind. Once you feel you have had enough and, hopefully, are nice and relaxed then stretch out your legs (they might be asleep), spread your fingers and stretch your arms, turn your head slowly to stretch your neck and get up. If you are nice and relaxed then try to maintain it for a while, perhaps with a cup of tea, a wander in the garden or just sitting quietly reading. If you have children then this isn't going to happen so wait until they are in bed or at school to find your quiet time.

Children are very good at meditation by the way. If your children are pre-schoolers they love to sit cross-legged with hands on knees and eyes closed. Once you get them in this position then quietly tell them a story, preferably one with imaginary creatures. The favourite one for my preschool Yoga classes was having them imagine they are climbing a huge big tree and at the top of the tree was a land of fairies who taught them to fly back to the ground. Make it up as you go along but nothing scary. Five minutes is long enough for the littlies. Next is the primary school children. They are happy to be led through the breathing technique then have them imagine they are flying. You need to speak quietly and slowly so your voice becomes their background. Tell them their arms become wings and the body becomes covered in feathers and they are on an air current floating across the sky. Don't forget to bring them slowly back to earth before opening their eyes and finishing. Up to 10 minutes maximum though. Once they are teens, even at 13, they are able to do the same as adults. So, if you have children then why not try it out. They will benefit and you get to spend that 10 minutes with quiet children!

Relaxation meditation can be done anywhere once you get used to it. If you drive around a lot in your job then when you stop for a coffee break find a park or other quiet place, lock the doors of the car and sit in it for 5 minutes with your eyes closed and just follow your breath. If someone comes along they will just think you are asleep, the locked doors will stop anyone annoying you. Trust me, I had a job that put me in such a position and this is how I used to get through the afternoon. Lunch then 5 minutes meditation. Starting the day with a 5 minute meditation before you get out of bed in the morning can do wonders for the day too. Just sit up when you wake and go from there. It works.

Your journey in meditation is a life long one, not a fad to try and throw away. You will find it useful throughout your life and it is especially important during times of stress, mental, emotional and physical. To be able to just turn inside for 10 minutes or more is one of the greatest medications you can give yourself – and it's free and always available. So get practising but please remember, it doesn't always happen straight away. Like anything that is good for you it takes practice and time to be able to achieve it naturally.

CHAPTER SIX

WALKING

MEDITATION

You may have come across the practise of walking meditation, usually connected to some kind of maze or other pattern on the ground. The idea of this is that you concentrate on where your feet are going and shut off the outside world. As there are wonderful places you can go to learn and experience this I am not going to dwell on the different kinds. However, you can practise a simple version in your own garden. Rather than try to mark out a complicated pattern simply walk up and down a particular path. For instance, if you have a rectangle lawn area then start at one corner and walk to the other side of the garden, take one or two paces to the side, turn around and walk back across the garden. Continue this pattern until you have covered the entire space (or a part of it if you have a large garden). During this time you just breath in and out gently and watch your feet. Don't think of anything. Once you have done this once or twice you might like to chant a mantra as you go. It is nice if you can hold your hands in prayer position in front of your heart to centre your thoughts but it is not necessary. If you are lucky enough to have the space to do so then perhaps a dedicated space in the garden can be made into a spiral using pavers or bricks with something in the centre like a bowl of crystals that can be the focal point to head towards. Make sure the spaces along the spiral are such that you can comfortably walk around towards the centre. If you are living in a space where none of this is possible then I have a friend who has a "portable" one, drawn on a large sheet of canvas that can be placed on the ground when needed. Brilliant idea Wendi.

So experiment, find your space and try walking meditation.

CHAPTER SEVEN

OTHER KINDS OF

MEDITATION

Most people these days are aware that Meditation aids relaxation, either practised on our own or in a group. However there are many different types of meditation that give different results to the practitioner and the following may give you insight as to how you can personally use meditation to make changes in your life.

Although many people have religious beliefs there are many also who would like to follow a Spiritual path without becoming involved in organised religion. **SPIRITUAL MEDITATION** leads us along this path. However, those who are involved in a religious life will also enjoy this because they can put their own beliefs into play. What happens in your own heart and mind stays in your own heart and mind.

If you haven't heard of **MANIFESTATION MEDITATION** over the last 5 years you have probably been meditating on a mountain somewhere or too busy to bother with it. The Secret, The Secrets to Success and other amazing and wondrous ideals come down to the simply using our own mind to manifest what you really want in life. It's not rocket science, it is meditation. If you would like to bring something into your life then you might like to give this a go. Please keep in mind though that this is not about relaxation it is about bringing something into your life that you would like to achieve or experience.

The human brain is capable of many wonderful actions and one of these is the ability to heal the body through thought and intention. Meditation is in fact a "complimentary health" method. Using meditation alongside traditional or natural medicine it has been proved to have a very positive affect. **HEALING MEDITATION** is now widely accepted whereas it was once frowned upon by those who thought only modern medicine could heal the sick. Now it is commonly used for healing and is often prescribed by a modern GP. As relaxing aids any kind of healing just the simple methods covered in the beginning of this book will help without any professional help. However, there are also many natural therapists who use Healing Meditation as a major part of the healing process.

ASTRAL TRAVELLING – yes you read correctly, it is quite commonly practised. During the 1960s, 70s and 80s we were introduced to Astral Travelling. This is a technique that allows the practitioner to 'leave' their corporeal body and seem to be in another place and/or time. It is sometimes used to 'travel' back in time to a former life. More on that later.

CHAPTER EIGHT

QIGONG AND TAI CHI

Qigong is one of the ancient health exercises being practised throughout the world today. Along with Tai Chi, Qigong is often practised daily, and in China people can be seen in the parks or in the fields early in the morning doing this slow and easy exercise. Once you have learnt the principal movements then it is with you for life. Personally, I have been practising for over 30 years. I will honestly say that I can thank my Qigong practice as well as my Yoga practice for my good health.

Qigong can be particularly beneficial for such problems as asthma, arthritis, hypertension and can relieve headaches. It is also beneficial for many other health problems. Qigong can be practised by people with physical disabilities, and I personally have had a few disabled students who enjoyed Qigong in their own way, modifying the movements to suit their disabilities. It is also safe to practice during pregnancy, in fact I have been thanked for teaching my pregnant Yoga students the art of Qigong because they can continue doing their practice even when their Yoga has to take a back seat.

In ancient times in China the peasants who had been working all day in the fields would come home to the cool of the evening and the moon became their "friend" whereas the Sun was beating down on them all day. As a result the Chinese would follow the moon times and use the cool evenings to wind down and relax. They were aware that from the day in the sun their bodies had heat, like steam, rising through them. They would feel this steam moving through their legs, arms and body. They also realised that this steam rising and falling through the body was related to their breathing patterns. After noting this feeling and the reaction of the body over a period of time they eventually discovered that each person had an energy centre and this was just below the naval. This centre made the body feel warm and strong and they called it the DANTIEN. With continued observation they found that this "steam" flow made the body warm and would also seem to be connected to their spirit or feeling of well-being. After a while it was discovered that the body had channels linking the organs of the body and there was also certain points along this channel that could be touched or massaged and this would affect the body organs. This energy that moved along the channels was called Qi (Chi) and so the Chinese method of acupuncture was developed.

Tai Chi works in a similar way. The main difference is that in Qigong you usually stay in the same spot whereas Tai Chi movements are more mobile. Please see if there are any classes in your area otherwise look on line. There are many wonderful videos available. Be aware though, learning Tai Chi from a video means that when you turn away from the screen you won't be able to see what the instructor is doing. One way to overcome this is to have a large mirror opposite the screen so you can see what you are supposed to be doing without getting a sore neck! Meanwhile, Qigong is done facing one way only and although the feet do a bit of moving you actually stay in the same direction. If you are over 50 and live in Australia then check out your local U3A classes because most of them offer Tai Chi and in some places it is free.

CHAPTER NINE

SPIRITUAL

MEDITATION

Most people think of Spiritual Meditation as prayer, however it is so much more than that. A prayer is often aimed towards a higher being in order to obtain some kind of assistance or to give thanks for that which has already happened. This is one form of Spiritual Meditation and it is important to many people. When you think of Spiritual Meditation do you see someone sitting in Lotus position with eyes closed in front of a statue of the Buddha or sitting in a church or other religious building with eyes closed in contemplation? Or do you see someone who seems to be "off with the fairies" as they sit on a hilltop? Well, they just might be practising Spiritual Meditation or they could just need some quiet time.

Spiritual Meditation is personal. Very personal. It is an opportunity to connect silently to a higher energy. This energy is most likely your own higher self, the part of you that is inside your very own being. If you like it could be the soul or the invisible seed that makes you who you are. It isn't the ego, that is the side of you that you want to show the world. It is further in than that. Imagine that there is a tiny radiant light somewhere inside you. The heart, the mind, the third eye. This is your inner being. It is what has been believed to be the light that switches off when you die or goes on to the next life if you believe in reincarnation. So, what has that got to do with meditation? It is everything to do with it. The outer world is there, where you can see it. Sometimes it gives you a hard time and sometimes it makes you laugh and sometimes it can be downright difficult to get on with. And it is in those moments that it is good to turn within and connect to the spiritual you, the inner you, the one that has always been there. It is not always easy to find but there is a way to try.

PRACTISE

Begin in your sacred space. The one you have for relaxation meditation. If you have a piece of Amethyst crystal then either place it in your hand or put it on your altar. If it is on a chain or leather then place it around your neck next to your skin. Amethyst connects you to your inner self. You will need to have complete privacy so make sure you try this when you are alone. Start by getting rid of the outside world by going back to the principals of the relaxation meditation and once you feel relaxed and closed off then close your eyes once more.

In the centre of your forehead between your eyebrows is the place referred to as the Third Eye. It is one of the major Chakras or energy centres of the human body and it can be very powerful. Now, with your mind on that Third Eye imagine you are in there, centred in the front of your mind and concentrate. You may begin to see a purple light, this is good but don't worry if you don't. After a while you need to let your mind go. Don't think, don't try to imagine anything, just be there and breath. After a while you may begin to feel another energy around you, this is good. Or you may 'see' in your mind's eye a form that could be a spiritual being. Some see the form of an Angel or a human figure surrounded by light. Others just feel amazing. I cannot tell you what you will see or feel as everyone is different but it will feel almost otherworldly.

Remember, this kind of meditation will not happen immediately. Some people practise relaxation meditation for years then all of a sudden they find they can go just that bit deeper and they feel they are on another level of being, a spiritual level. Others connect on the second or third try. It could be that your inner being is content as it is and there is no need to go any further. Some who have a religious belief might connect to their God or Goddess and others might see a loved one who has passed on. Even if you don't "get it" then you have spent some time in meditation and that is also a very good thing. The secret is – don't try too hard just let it happen

CHAPTER TEN

MANIFESTATION

MEDITATION

This is one of my favourites. I have used it frequently throughout my life and is usually works. The most important thing to remember, BE CAREFUL WHAT YOU ASK FOR because it might come back on you. Please, *never involve another person in your manifestation because you are not to meddle with someone else's destiny.* The first step is to come to a decision about what you would like to bring into your life. The following are some suggestions of what this kind of manifestation can bring about.

LOVE – always a good one and very popular.

MONEY – something most people would like more of.

A NEW CAR

YOUR OWN HOME

TRAVEL

A NEW START IN LIFE

WEIGHT LOSS OR GAIN

GOOD HEALTH

A NEW CAREER

There are many more reasons to want to use manifestation and they all come down to using the same method. First you must really want this because your intent is the most important part of the whole procedure. If you are into sport then perhaps you would like to be better. See yourself achieving your goal or if golf is your thing you may want to visualise a hole in one. Time to write down what you would like to bring into your life and be sure because you don't want the whole thing to backfire on your. It is always a good idea to start with something small and work up to the bigger things. I do know of someone who manifested "more time for relaxation" and ended up breaking a leg and staying home for 6 weeks. Yep, that was me. So, as I have said, be careful what you ask for or it could backfire. For this exercise we will start with "Good Health".

PRACTISE

Please begin by entering your Sacred Space and writing "I would like to have good health" (or something like that) down on a nice piece of paper that can be folded up after the meditation and stashed away. Now hold that piece of paper in your hand and settle in. Begin with some centring breaths and become comfortable. You might want to read this meditation onto a recording device of some kind so you can have it playing to help you do the meditation because you will need to practise a bit first.

Begin by taking several slow breaths while sitting comfortably in your sacred space. Close your eyes and just concentrate on your breathing. In through the nose and out through the nose (if you can). Allow the breath to flow naturally and turn your mind within. To do this just concentrate on your breathing and let the world go away for a while.

Imagine that you are walking slowly up a gentle slope. At the top of the slope you will see a type of temple or pagoda. When you reach the door open it and walk through closing the door behind you. Looking around you will see a well in the centre and four doors around the walls that are Yellow, Red, Blue and Green. You walk to the well in the centre and dip your hands in the water. This well is your life as it stands and all the things that you have experienced in your life are contained in the water of the well. Now walk to the first door, the Yellow door, and when you open it think of all the things in your life that make you happy. Perhaps it is family, friends, your home or some other part of your life now or in the past. Feel that happiness then turn to your right and walk to the Red door. The Red door represents the power and strength that is within you and when you open the door you will see a large sword point down waiting for you. This is your strength so reach in and take the sword. Hold it firmly in your hand, turn to the right and walk to the Blue Door. This door represents all your achievements in life. As you open the door there will be images of your achievements. Maybe a diploma or degree, a cruise ship representing a holiday you had, a car you saved up for, something you made with your own hands that you were very proud of. We all have something in our lives that remind us of what we are capable of, even small achievements. See something or many things that you have achieved and walk to the right to the Green door. The Green door is where you will ask for that which you wish to achieve. The green represents growth. Now is the time to ask for the Good Health you wish to bring in or retain within your life. One of the best ways to do this is to ask directly "I want my body and mind to be healthy and strong." Reach into the door and receive in your hand a scroll that is a report from a health check-up that gives you 100% and a picture of you looking strong and healthy. Now take that scroll and picture to the well and drop them in, allowing them to sink into the water and become part of you. Next you walk back to the Yellow door and giving thanks for the happiness in your life gently close the door and walk to the right to the Red door. Place the sword back and give thanks for the strength within your life, close the door and walk to the right.

At the Blue door give thanks for all the achievements in your life so far, close the door and walk to the right to the Green door. Give thanks for the Good Health you have just been given and close the Green door. Returning to the main door, leave the building, close the door behind you with a word or two of thanks and walk down the slope to finally bring yourself back to the present.

Once you open your eyes spend about 5 minutes in the peace and quiet of your Sacred Space then take the piece of paper and place it somewhere special to you. Perhaps you could leave it on your "Altar" under a crystal or you may have a box or other place you keep things. Now leave it there. Don't go back to it soon just trust the Universe to have listened.

Manifestation does not happen overnight. It may take a little while but I assure you it will happen if you let your life flow and don't force it. Obviously this meditation for Good Health won't work if you keep eating bad foods, smoke, take drugs and drink alcohol. You have to be responsible for some of the outcome and you can help it along by being aware of these bad habits. But don't be surprised if you begin to turn down offers to join friends who are doing those things and your visit to the supermarket might have you wandering through the fruit and vegetables rather than the junk food sections. You might get the urge to join a Gym or Yoga class or go for a morning walk when you didn't before. You do have to put in some effort you know but the urges in your mind to do these healthy things are the result of your manifestation. This meditation can be used for any manifestation, just change what you ask for at the Green door and 'receive' something that represents what you are asking for, such as a car, house etc.

Another way you can use Manifestation is, as I said earlier, while being involved in sport. Let's say you are involved in archery. Your ideal result would probably be a bullseye. When you are standing there, bow in hand and arrow at the ready, the target is out there in front of you and you would like the arrow to go straight to the target. Close your eyes for a moment and breathe. In your mind see the target and see the arrow going straight to the centre and hitting the bullseye. Now softly open your eyes and let the arrow go. The same can be done with golf or any other sport that requires you to hit a target and gives you that quiet opportunity to manifest the result. Try it, you just never know.

CHAPTER ELEVEN

HEALING

MEDITATION

In the last chapter I covered using Manifestation Meditation to achieve a healthy body and mind. However, if you have a health problem, or someone close to you has, then you may like to try a Healing Meditation. The great thing about this is the fact that it doesn't interfere with medication or other treatments. You are using your mind to heal your body and/or mind. The brain is a wonderful thing in so far as you are what you think you are and we have been told for a few decades now that the Power of Positive Thinking can make incredible changes in our lives. It doesn't mean that you can sit down today with a broken arm, think it healed and the next day it is. What it means is that over a period of time you 'convince' your body to heal. The meditation should be personalised to your or your loved one's condition. You will need to be clear on what you want to achieve and it doesn't hurt to write that down to clarify. There are many conditions that can be helped with meditation, although you still have to allow the body or mind to heal in a natural time.

PRACTISE

Begin by entering your Sacred Space. However, if you are in hospital or somewhere away from home then you will just need a quiet place so you won't be interrupted. This can also be done sitting in a church, chapel, temple or mosque where you can be left alone and it will also be a spiritual place. You don't need to be religious to sit quietly in one of those places and if the Priest or other comes to see what you are there for just tell them you need some quiet time to contemplate. You don't need to say more than that. Thank them for caring and let them understand you wish to be left alone.

You are going to spend about 10 minutes getting into the state you need to be in by sitting peacefully and following the flow of your breath – the same applies to all these meditations. Once you feel comfortable and relaxed you need to think of your problem, don't worry about it or try to 'fix' it, just have it in your mind. There are a few ways of doing this but I find the best is the White Light manifestation. Imagine in your mind a bright white light surrounding your body, take your time here. The light needs to surround you, fill out your Aura – that energy we all have around our bodies. Once you are surrounded by that white energy imagine it is entering your body through your skin until your whole body is full of white light energy. Now you find the part of you that needs healing and see that area filled with purple or mauve energy – this is the healing energy – and allow it to be absorbed into the part of you that needs healing. At this stage, if you wish to, you can call upon any deity, angel, higher being or other to come into you and heal you. If you do not wish to do this then just allow that purple energy to do the job. In your mind you can think the following: "My body is healthy and strong. My mind is healthy and strong. I am healing and becoming well." Or words to that effect and repeat it over and over for a while. Once you feel that you have been there long enough (trust yourself here) then you go back to your breathing for a while, gently open your eyes and stay put for a couple of minutes.

This is a good general healing meditation. If you are doing it for another person then you see them within your mind and see the white light then the purple one within their body. They do not need to be there and this is called 'absent healing'. It's very like when a group of people get together in a place of worship and do healing prayers. The power of the mind whether singularly or in a group is an amazing thing and very strong. It's not so much the deity or other that is being called upon, it is more the energy a group of people put out there that does the job.

You can also use this Healing Meditation to heal an animal that you care about and I believe it could be used on any natural life, although I have never tried that myself.

CRYSTAL HEALING MEDITATION

Using crystals to aid healing is another form of healing meditation. The idea is to find the right crystal for the particular problem and use it during your meditation. There is a lot of information available on which crystals effect which part of the body and mind. If you have a health problem then it is always advisable to seek professional advice before going down this path as the problem you are experiencing may be a sign of something else. However, there are many crystals that are very safe to use for general healing. One of the best is Clear Quartz as it can be a stand in for many other crystals. I am going to concentrate on the balancing healing meditation that I often do myself and it will help to bring on general health and healing. Working on the Chakras, the energy centres of the body, we can bring balance to the body and allow it to continue healing itself from imbalance. So, in order to do this is is best to do it lying down. I have a very comfortable carpet in my healing space that I can lie on or you can do this in bed – falling asleep is sometimes a result here, although this is sometimes what your body requires at that moment. So, find your quiet place, prepare the room to be comfortable temperature wise and gather up what you need. This is not always best done outside because you may be so very comfortable lying there and at the very moment you are about to get into your zone an insect lands on your nose – in which case you need to start from the beginning. So, best done indoors or in a screened space.

You will need – something comfortable to lie on – if it is cool then a light covering will help; Some meditative music in the background is nice; Peace and quiet away from other people and animals and of course, crystals. The best ones to use for this kind of balancing meditation are easily available. First of all *make sure you have cleansed the crystals.* To do this I like to wash them in salt water (no you don't need to go to the beach, just salt in rain or spring water will do) and either leave them in the sun all day or in the moon overnight. There are some who use incense smoke to cleanse, whatever is right for you. Once they are cleansed then keep them in a nice cotton bag or a container for future use. If you don't know anything about Chakras there are many throughout the body, however, for this practise I use the seven from the Crown through to the Base and they are as follows. The Crown chakra is located right on the top of your head, somewhere near the fontanelle (soft spot on a baby's head). The Third Eye chakra is located behind the bridge of the nose between the eyes. The Throat chakra is behind that little indent at the base of your throat. The Heart chakra is not over your heart but in the centre of your chest. The Solar Plexus chakra is about a hand width above your navel. The Sacral chakra is the same distance below your navel and finally the Base chakra is virtually up between your legs but we use the area over the pubic hair to make things a little easier. I have used the English words for this because many have problems with the Hindi pronunciation that is commonly used. Now the crystals I am going to suggest are the easy ones to get hold of and please don't think big is best, it will be very hard to balance a great chunk of crystal on some parts of your body.

Crown   Clear quartz (big as you like because it can sit on the floor above your head)

Third Eye   Amethyst (not too big it has to sit on your forehead between your eyes)

Throat   Aquamarine (or something else light blue)

Heart   Either Rose quartz or Jade (green and pink both work here)

Solar Plexus   Tiger Eye

Sacral   Carnelian or some other orange/yellow crystal

Base   Obsidian

On top of these four more Obsidian crystals can be used on both the hands and below the feet but this is not necessary at this stage.

PRACTISE

Have your stones beside you where you can reach down and pick them up without sitting up. Lie down on the floor or bed. Relax for a few minutes to rid yourself of the world outside and place the Clear quarts on the floor above your head. Now, place the Obsidian on your body (fully dressed is OK) just above the pubic area, next the Carnelian on your

Sacral area, up to the Solar Plexus and place the Tiger Eye and so on up the body until all the stones are in place. Take a few centring breaths and allow your mind to go the Base chakra area. Try to see the black stone there in your mind and concentrate upon it. Keep your mind there for a while then finish by thinking or saying out loud "I am grounded" 3 times. Leave that there and bring your mind up to the Sacral stone. Do the same here, centring your mind on the stone then finish by saying "I am strong in body and mind" 3 times. Keep going up – at the Solar Plexus the words are "I am happy most of the time" 3 times, the Heart is "I am open to give and receive love" 3 times, the Throat "I say what I mean and mean what I say" 3 times, the Third Eye "I am true to myself" 3 times and finally the Crown "I am connected and part of the Universe" 3 times. These statements might seen to have no connection to your health, mental or physical, however, keep in mind that if your mind and spirit are in good balance then your body will follow. It might sound simplified but it really is that simple. Ill health will grow in a body or mind that is out of balance. And, guess what, none of this will hurt you at all.

So try it and when you get this right you might like to find some information on healing specific problems with meditation and crystals but if you haven't done this before then start simple and work your way up. The series of books called The Crystal Bible are definitely worth a look for this information.

CHAPTER TWELVE

ASTRAL TRAVELLING

I first learned about Astral Travelling in the 1980s when it was one of the New Age things you did with a group of other like minded people. I don't know how many actually achieved it but I felt amazing when I had my first experience. It is not something that is easily described but if you manage it then you will never forget it.

PRACTISE

You begin with the normal breath work in a quiet place. Make sure you are not going to be disturbed and also make sure that there are no electronic items in the room or it will interfere with the results. You will need to connect with the Universe to achieve any result and this is something that is very difficult for beginners or those with preconceived ideas on the subject. Allow your mind to be free of what you think should happen and just wait for it. The deeper your meditation becomes over a time then the more likely you will be able to do this, however there are beginners who have achieve the experience on the first go. If you come across a group that is doing it then please join in if you can and if it doesn't cost you money. (Yes there are people taking advantage of beginners! You know that of course don't you?)

An easy way to try it out is as follows:

Settle in with your breath work and stay quiet for about 5 to 10 minutes just closing off the outside world. Once your mind is clear try to imagine a white or golden light, like a thick rope, coming from the top of your head – think Crown Chakra. Gradually extend this light out into the universe (or space) until you find yourself away from the Earth and into space. Once you are there think of yourself floating off away from the Earth and allow yourself to just travel. I cannot tell you what you see because everyone experiences it in a different way. When you think it is time then travel back down your "rope" until you feel you are back inside your body, follow your breath for a while until you feel ready then gently open your eyes behind your hands, dry washing the eyes then release them. Please try to keep peaceful for the rest of the day because if you have achieved Astral Travel then your body and mind may be tired. A cup of your favourite relaxing herbal tea is the best follow-up. Good luck with this one. It can be beautiful. If nothing happens don't worry, it might the next time.

The other way that is sometimes referred to as Astral Travel is 'hovering' just above your physical body. It can be best to lie down to do this one but not necessary. Just make sure you aren't going to drop off to sleep. Even if you do it means your body needed to so try again when you wake up. Now, same as before. Go into your Sacred Space and begin with your breath work. Take your time. Then you need to relax the body so there is no tension. Start with your feet, tense and relax with your breath. Breathe in tense – breathe out relax. Then work your way up your body one section at a time until you reach your skull where you screw up your face and head and release it. Now go back to your breath for a bit. Once you feel totally relaxed you need to visualise your body surrounded by the white or purple light, just filling your aura. When this feels right you imagine that your inner body is beginning to float away from your physical body, slowly and peacefully. The inner body is now floating just above your physical body and that's where you stay. Completely separate but joined to the body by the light surrounding your physical body. It sounds strange and when you first experience it you may want to stay there forever but you can't. When you have been floating for a while allow your inner body to gently float down back into the physical, take as long as you like following your breathing and when you are ready just gently open your eyes and stay there for a bit. Don't rush this, so don't do it if you need to be somewhere else or if you have chores to finish. Follow it up with a nice cup of Chamomile or other calming tea. If it doesn't work the first time don't worry, try again in a few days or the next week. Not everyone can achieve Astral Travelling but it is definitely worth a try.

CHAPTER THIRTEEN

RELAXATION AT

WORK

The following are short exercises dealing with **Office Tension and Stiff Muscles**, they can also be used during the day at work to relieve the body of the physical stress involved in working with people. Each one should be done 3 times. This is not a meditation, just a way to relax body and mind.

Link your hands together, palms away from your body and arms straight out in front of your chest. Breathe in pushing away, hold for a couple of breaths then relax.

Link your hands together behind your chair (or back), lift your arms slightly, breathe in and push away from the body, hold for a couple of breaths then relax.

Take arms straight out to the sides (level with shoulders) palms turned out, stretch out. Flex hands down then on exhale bring hands back to knees.

Stretch arms up and "press the ceiling", hold for a few breaths then relax.

Reach up behind your back with one hand and down from the top with the other, holding hands with yourself if you can, hold for a few breaths then relax.(hold a ruler between your hands if you can't reach.

Push the chair away from your desk. Breathe in, raise the body up then breathing out reach down and clasp your ankles, letting your head drop loosely. Arch the head up looking towards the ceiling then relax. Come up slowly to sitting.

Lift one leg – keeping it straight – flex the foot towards the body, hold then lower (do the same on the other side)

Keeping the body facing forward, slowly turn your head to the left, then the right, then up and down – very slowly or you can "wrench" the neck muscles.

Close your eyes for a few minutes and breathe gently trying not to think of anything.

It is very important that you endeavour to walk away from work for 10 – 30 minutes each day. There is a very sound theory that your mind can only work efficiently for 4 hours at a time then it loses the ability to continue with 100% efficiency. After a break it begins to work once more. Imagine your mind is like a computer. You need to back it up now and then so try to think of your 10-30 minute break as your brain doing a backup. There a many reasons why it is important to remember this, one of which is making sure you don't suffer from burnout. Taking a short break will allow your mind to settle and enable you to think and operate in a more productive way. If you are working with the public it can be very tiring as you are also taking on their stress on top of any you may have accumulated yourself. By allowing this to "drain away" for a while you are physically and mentally ready for the rest of the day.

It is also very important that you "leave work at work". Closing the door on work when you leave in the afternoon can be a physical act that will trigger a mental reaction. The easiest way is to turn and face the outside of your workplace as you leave and actually (silently) say "good-bye" to the building. If you travel by car then as you enter the car your thoughts should be on driving the car, not work. If you travel by public transport then perhaps you can do a crossword puzzle or read a book, anything except thinking of work while you travel home. When you reach home, turn off all outside thoughts of work or driving and concentrate on your home life. People who run their own business will have the most trouble doing this. It is so easy to get home and sit down on the computer to get more work done. If you have to do this remember to give yourself a time limit. The healthiest time to eat a meal in the evening is between 5.00 and 7.00pm so make this your break. If you are the cook then even better. There is nothing like cooking to take your mind away from other tasks – it is very good for the mind, body and soul.

By physically and mentally dividing our life into sections we are able to concentrate on the job at hand rather than what has or will happen in a different phase of our lives. The reverse is also true, if you have problems at home then that is where they should be. If needs be then you can organise a Counsellor to discuss these problems with, not your workmates who may also have enough of their own. However, the old fashioned way of dealing with stress was to sit around the kitchen table with a coffee or tea and discuss it with mum or grandma or your best friend. If you are lucky enough to be able to do this then go for it. Apart from being able to understand your life it's free!!! Perhaps you can take a nice cake with you as an appreciation. Another great way to relax is to go and watch, or take part in, sport. Saturday afternoon sitting watching a cricket match, a football game or other sport is very good for relaxation.

PROLOGUE

To many people sitting doing nothing is wasting time. According to some beliefs we are born with so many breaths and in others we are born to achieve something. Perhaps we were born to just live the current life as best we can.

It doesn't matter what your beliefs are it is more important that you make the most of the life you are living at this moment. From the time we are born until the time we die it is more important to face the daily challenges in the best frame of mind that we can or it is just decades of wasting time.

When we rise in the morning after sleep most people will begin by thinking of what the day is for. Work, school, personal achievements or just lazing about. Whatever the day has in store it is important to approach it in the best frame of mind possible in order to achieve results. If your mind is constantly working on what will be happening tomorrow, the next month or the next year then how is it possible to concentrate on what needs to be achieved today? Simply by giving your mind a break sometime during the day then you give it a chance to concentrate on what it needs to do next. Little grabs of "time out" for your mind are just as important as a 30 minute meditation. However, that 30 minute meditation gives the mind a chance to reset. Once a day, three times a week or just once a week on Sunday morning, it doesn't matter, it still gives your mind a good break from thinking. Calming that Monkey Mind allows you to face the next challenge life has to offer.

Remember, many good things can happen by just sitting still quietly, doing nothing. Over a very long time we have been conditioned to believe that the only way to improve our quality of life is by working harder and putting more effort into doing more things. Meditation is not doing, it is effortless and in fact you cannot "do" meditation you can only relax and flow into it, allow it to happen. Surrendering to your inner self relinquishes the compulsive urges that drive us into constant thought. Without a relaxed mind we can never totally relax the body. Time to stop "doing" all the time, just sit down and breathe.

Om Shanti

ABOUT THE AUTHOR

Living in a quiet Eco Village in Central Queensland, Australia has given Heather the time and energy to follow up on ideas that have been in the melting pot for many years. As a Freelance Journalist there was the satisfaction of letting readers know what was happening, however her storytelling gift was finally realised with the release of Under Her Protection in 2020 and Finding Bicycles in 2021. The decision to leave fiction behind for a while and concentrate on imparting decades of knowledge was the next step. Following 23 years teaching Yoga, meditation and Qigong it was time to retire from physical teaching and put all that knowledge into print to allow those who cannot attend physical classes, for many reasons, to take a step towards something new and wonderful. It does not mean the fiction has been forgotten, just moved aside for a while.

BY THE SAME AUTHOR

(Available in either hard copy or digital)

UNDER HER PROTECTION – Published 2020 (Fiction)

In a future following the Climate Catastrophe that changed the Earth forever, a gang of marauders are terrorising the people on the Plains of Parlat. Nothing has been able to stop them until a local Wise Woman decides enough is enough and with the help of others sets about to be rid of them once and for all. Good natural magic and a bit of help from a surprising source finally solves the problem.

FINDING BICYCLES – Published 2021 (Fiction)

In a future many years following the collapse of the technical age and a return of many societies to the simple ways of the Middle Ages, Rosalind will tell you the story as she lives her life between being a member of a community of women who follow the ways of the Earth Mother and the avid traveller seeing the world with her father. From a rather precarious event as a young girl on her way to be married to learning the ways to heal and teach nature's ways she occasionally escapes to the high seas with her father and discovers that not all the world has lost the technology and lifestyles that she believed disappeared with the Great Climate Catastrophe.

GUIDE TO THE NEW AGE - Searching for Self

Ancient Wisdom for the 21st Century

- Published 2022 (Non fiction)

In a world where we are told anything is possible it can be a very confusing place for someone who is just trying to improve their way of life. Searching for Self may help you to decide just what it is that you need to change in your life or perhaps you will find that you don't need to change anything at all, just look at life differently. Ancient Wisdom for the 21st Century may guide you through the maze of New Age ideas and ancient practices that are available. From the 1960s when we began to open our minds to many ideas that were hidden for a very long time to the 21st century where we are able to search on line for so many wondrous ideas, old and new. I hope this may help your journey